Dedication

This planner is dedicated to physicians of all specialties. Thank you for your work and dedication to the patients that you serve. In particular, to my brother Dr. Juan Flores. You have always been available during every family medical 'crisis.' Thank you for your support, kindness and patience.

Maria A. Flores

THIS BOOK
BELONGS TO:

Physician's Notes

MONTHLY
PLANNER

The Inspiring Journal (2022, November 3). Motivational quotes by famous people.
www.theinspiringjournal.com

Touch the Heart, Reach the Soul, LLC
Maria Flores
Author, Founder

Inspirational faith based journals, notebooks, books, artwork
and gift items.
https://touchtheheartreachthesoul.com
https://touchtheheartreachthesoul.store
customerservice@touchtheheartreachthesoul.com

JANUARY

SIDE NOTE	MONDAY	TUESDAY	WEDNESDAY

THURSDAY	FRIDAY	SATURDAY	SUNDAY

"The secret of getting ahead is getting started" Mark Twain

WEEKLY PLANNER

Priorities

Monday

Tuesday

Wednesday

Notes

Thursday

Friday

Saturday

Sunday

WEEKLY PLANNER

Priorities

Monday

Tuesday

Wednesday

Notes

Thursday

Friday

Saturday

Sunday

WEEKLY PLANNER

Priorities

Monday

Tuesday

Wednesday

Notes

Thursday

Friday

Saturday

Sunday

WEEKLY PLANNER

Priorities

Monday

Tuesday

Wednesday

Notes

Thursday

Friday

Saturday

Sunday

FEBRUARY

SIDE NOTE	MONDAY	TUESDAY	WEDNESDAY

THURSDAY	FRIDAY	SATURDAY	SUNDAY

“The best revenge is massive success.” Frank Sinatra

WEEKLY PLANNER

Priorities

Monday

Tuesday

Wednesday

Notes

Thursday

Friday

Saturday

Sunday

WEEKLY PLANNER

Priorities

Monday

Tuesday

Wednesday

Notes

Thursday

Friday

Saturday

Sunday

WEEKLY PLANNER

Priorities

Monday

Tuesday

Wednesday

Notes

Thursday

Friday

Saturday

Sunday

WEEKLY PLANNER

Priorities

Monday

Tuesday

Wednesday

Notes

Thursday

Friday

Saturday

Sunday

MARCH

SIDE NOTE	MONDAY	TUESDAY	WEDNESDAY

THURSDAY	FRIDAY	SATURDAY	SUNDAY

‘I have not failed. I’ve just found 10,000 ways that won’t work.” Thomas Edison

WEEKLY PLANNER

Priorities

Monday

Tuesday

Wednesday

Notes

Thursday

Friday

Saturday

Sunday

WEEKLY PLANNER

Priorities

Monday

Tuesday

Wednesday

Notes

Thursday

Friday

Saturday

Sunday

WEEKLY PLANNER

Priorities

Monday

Tuesday

Wednesday

Notes

Thursday

Friday

Saturday

Sunday

WEEKLY PLANNER

Priorities

Monday

Tuesday

Wednesday

Notes

Thursday

Friday

Saturday

Sunday

APRIL

SIDE NOTE	MONDAY	TUESDAY	WEDNESDAY

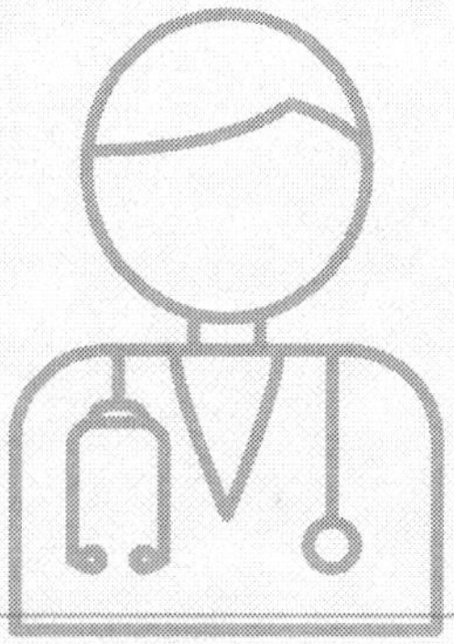

THURSDAY	FRIDAY	SATURDAY	SUNDAY
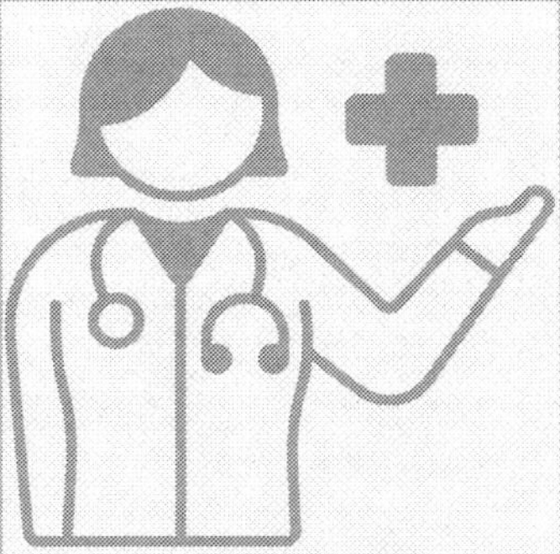			

"Build your own dreams, or someone else will hire you to build theirs." Farrah Gray

WEEKLY PLANNER

Priorities

Monday

Tuesday

Wednesday

Notes

Thursday

Friday

Saturday

Sunday

WEEKLY PLANNER

Priorities

Monday

Tuesday

Wednesday

Notes

Thursday

Friday

Saturday

Sunday

WEEKLY PLANNER

Priorities

Monday

Tuesday

Wednesday

Notes

Thursday

Friday

Saturday

Sunday

WEEKLY PLANNER

Priorities

Monday

Tuesday

Wednesday

Notes

Thursday

Friday

Saturday

Sunday

MAY

SIDE NOTE	MONDAY	TUESDAY	WEDNESDAY

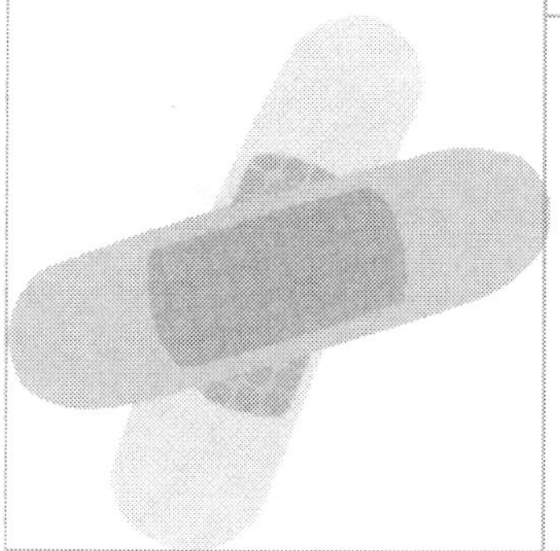

THURSDAY	FRIDAY	SATURDAY	SUNDAY

"It's never too late to be what you might have been." George Eliot

WEEKLY PLANNER

Priorities

Monday

Tuesday

Wednesday

Notes

Thursday

Friday

Saturday

Sunday

WEEKLY PLANNER

Priorities

Monday

Tuesday

Wednesday

Notes

Thursday

Friday

Saturday

Sunday

WEEKLY PLANNER

Priorities

Monday

Tuesday

Wednesday

Notes

Thursday

Friday

Saturday

Sunday

WEEKLY PLANNER

Priorities

Monday

Tuesday

Wednesday

Notes

Thursday

Friday

Saturday

Sunday

JUNE

SIDE NOTE

MONDAY	TUESDAY	WEDNESDAY

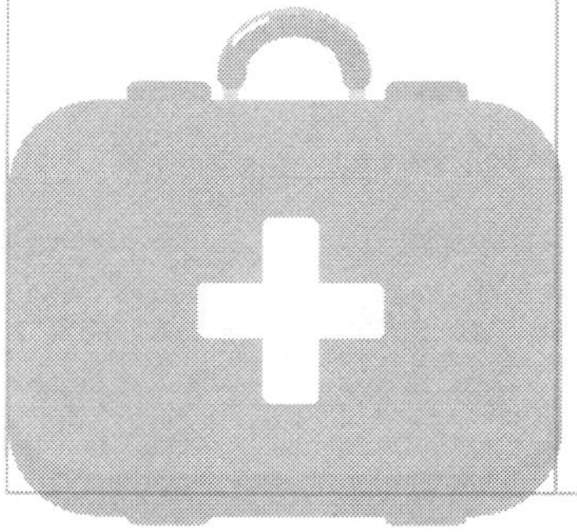

THURSDAY	FRIDAY	SATURDAY	SUNDAY

"Nothing happens unless first a dream." Carl Sandburg

WEEKLY PLANNER

Priorities

Monday

Tuesday

Wednesday

Notes

Thursday

Friday

Saturday

Sunday

WEEKLY PLANNER

Priorities

Monday

Tuesday

Wednesday

Notes

Thursday

Friday

Saturday

Sunday

WEEKLY PLANNER

Priorities

Monday

Tuesday

Wednesday

Notes

Thursday

Friday

Saturday

Sunday

WEEKLY PLANNER

Priorities

Monday

Tuesday

Wednesday

Notes

Thursday

Friday

Saturday

Sunday

JULY

SIDE NOTE	MONDAY	TUESDAY	WEDNESDAY

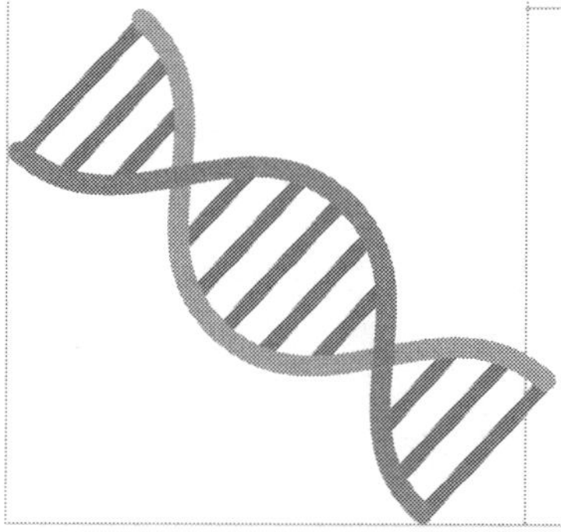

THURSDAY	FRIDAY	SATURDAY	SUNDAY

“Don’t limit yourself.” Mary Kay Ash

WEEKLY PLANNER

Priorities

Monday

Tuesday

Wednesday

Notes

Thursday

Friday

Saturday

Sunday

WEEKLY PLANNER

Priorities

Monday

Tuesday

Wednesday

Notes

Thursday

Friday

Saturday

Sunday

WEEKLY PLANNER

Priorities

Monday

Tuesday

Wednesday

Notes

Thursday

Friday

Saturday

Sunday

WEEKLY PLANNER

Priorities

Monday

Tuesday

Wednesday

Notes

Thursday

Friday

Saturday

Sunday

AUGUST

SIDE NOTE	MONDAY	TUESDAY	WEDNESDAY

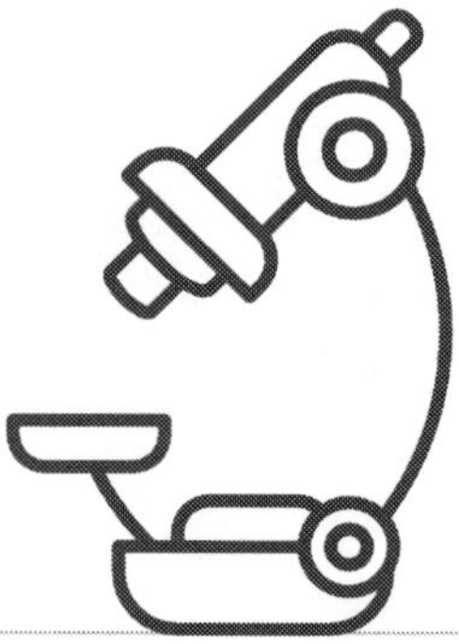

THURSDAY	FRIDAY	SATURDAY	SUNDAY

"Either write something worth reading or do something worth writing." Benjamin Franklin

WEEKLY PLANNER

Priorities

Monday

Tuesday

Wednesday

Notes

Thursday

Friday

Saturday

Sunday

WEEKLY PLANNER

Priorities

Monday

Tuesday

Wednesday

Notes

Thursday

Friday

Saturday

Sunday

WEEKLY PLANNER

Priorities

Monday

Tuesday

Wednesday

Notes

Thursday

Friday

Saturday

Sunday

WEEKLY PLANNER

Priorities

Monday

Tuesday

Wednesday

Notes

Thursday

Friday

Saturday

Sunday

SEPTEMBER

SIDE NOTE	MONDAY	TUESDAY	WEDNESDAY

THURSDAY	FRIDAY	SATURDAY	SUNDAY

“Every man dies. Not every man really lives.” William Wallace

WEEKLY PLANNER

Priorities

Monday

Tuesday

Wednesday

Notes

Thursday

Friday

Saturday

Sunday

WEEKLY PLANNER

Priorities

Monday

Tuesday

Wednesday

Notes

Thursday

Friday

Saturday

Sunday

WEEKLY PLANNER

Priorities

Monday

Tuesday

Wednesday

Notes

Thursday

Friday

Saturday

Sunday

WEEKLY PLANNER

Priorities

Monday

Tuesday

Wednesday

Notes

Thursday

Friday

Saturday

Sunday

OCTOBER

SIDE NOTE	MONDAY	TUESDAY	WEDNESDAY
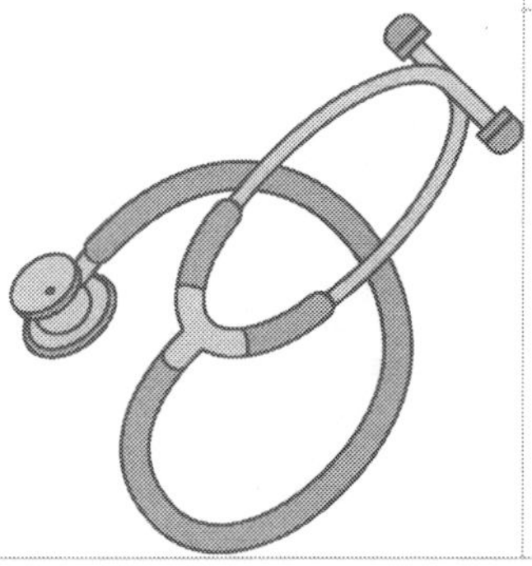			

THURSDAY	FRIDAY	SATURDAY	SUNDAY

“Men who know exactly what they want of life, do not stop wishing.” Andrew Carnegie

WEEKLY PLANNER

Priorities

Monday

Tuesday

Wednesday

Notes

Thursday

Friday

Saturday

Sunday

WEEKLY PLANNER

Priorities

Monday

Tuesday

Wednesday

Notes

Thursday

Friday

Saturday

Sunday

WEEKLY PLANNER

Priorities

Monday

Tuesday

Wednesday

Notes

Thursday

Friday

Saturday

Sunday

WEEKLY PLANNER

Priorities

Monday

Tuesday

Wednesday

Notes

Thursday

Friday

Saturday

Sunday

NOVEMBER

SIDE NOTE	MONDAY	TUESDAY	WEDNESDAY

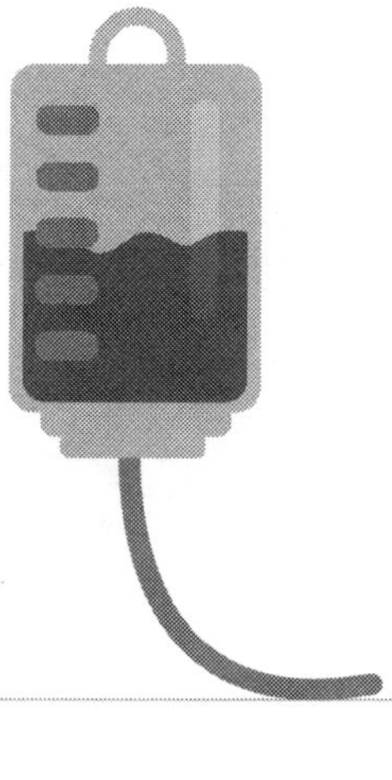

THURSDAY	FRIDAY	SATURDAY	SUNDAY

"Touch times never last, but tough people do." Robert Schuller

WEEKLY PLANNER

Priorities

Monday

Tuesday

Wednesday

Notes

Thursday

Friday

Saturday

Sunday

WEEKLY PLANNER

Priorities

Monday

Tuesday

Wednesday

Notes

Thursday

Friday

Saturday

Sunday

WEEKLY PLANNER

Priorities

Monday

Tuesday

Wednesday

Notes

Thursday

Friday

Saturday

Sunday

WEEKLY PLANNER

Priorities

Monday

Tuesday

Wednesday

Notes

Thursday

Friday

Saturday

Sunday

DECEMBER

SIDE NOTE	MONDAY	TUESDAY	WEDNESDAY

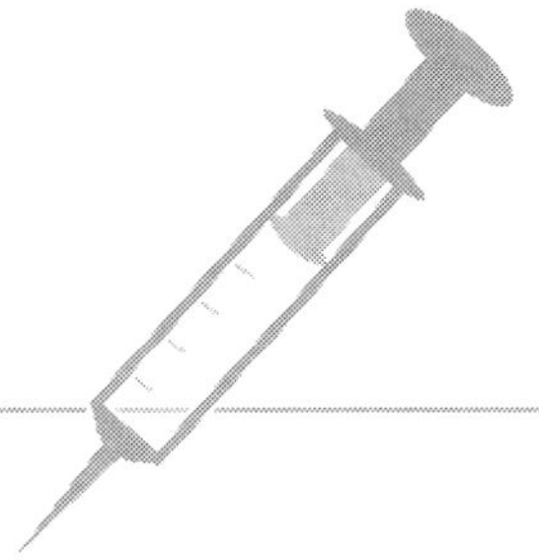

THURSDAY	FRIDAY	SATURDAY	SUNDAY

"Discontent is the first necessity of progress." Thomas Edison

WEEKLY PLANNER

Priorities

Monday

Tuesday

Wednesday

Notes

Thursday

Friday

Saturday

Sunday

WEEKLY PLANNER

Priorities

Monday

Tuesday

Wednesday

Notes

Thursday

Friday

Saturday

Sunday

WEEKLY PLANNER

Priorities

Monday

Tuesday

Wednesday

Notes

Thursday

Friday

Saturday

Sunday

WEEKLY PLANNER

Priorities

Monday

Tuesday

Wednesday

Notes

Thursday

Friday

Saturday

Sunday

TO DO LIST

DATE:

TO DO LIST

DATE:

TO DO LIST

DATE:

TO DO LIST

DATE:

TO DO LIST

DATE:

TO DO LIST

DATE:

TO DO LIST

DATE:

TO DO LIST

DATE:

TO DO LIST

DATE:

TO DO LIST

DATE:

NOTES:

NOTES:

NOTES:

NOTES:

NOTES:

NOTES:

NOTES:

NOTES:

NOTES:

NOTES:

Conferences

Conferences

Conferences

Conferences

Conferences

VACATION

VACATION

VACATION

VACATION

VACATION

VACATION

CONTINUING EDUCATION

CONTINUING EDUCATION

CONTINUING EDUCATION

		☐ ___ ☐ ___ ☐ ___
		☐ ___ ☐ ___ ☐ ___
		☐ ___ ☐ ___ ☐ ___
		☐ ___ ☐ ___ ☐ ___
		☐ ___ ☐ ___ ☐ ___
		☐ ___ ☐ ___ ☐ ___
		☐ ___ ☐ ___ ☐ ___

CONTINUING EDUCATION

CONTINUING EDUCATION

CONTINUING EDUCATION

IMPORTANT CONTACTS

Name
Phone
Email
Address

Name
Phone
Email
Address

Name
Phone
Email
Address

Name
Phone
Email
Address

Name
Phone
Email
Address

Name
Phone
Email
Address

Name
Phone
Email
Address

Name
Phone
Email
Address

IMPORTANT CONTACTS

Name

Phone

Email

Address

Name

Phone

Email

Address

Name

Phone

Email

Address

Name

Phone

Email

Address

Name

Phone

Email

Address

Name

Phone

Email

Address

Name

Phone

Email

Address

Name

Phone

Email

Address

IMPORTANT CONTACTS

Name
Phone
Email
Address

Name
Phone
Email
Address

Name
Phone
Email
Address

Name
Phone
Email
Address

Name
Phone
Email
Address

Name
Phone
Email
Address

Name
Phone
Email
Address

Name
Phone
Email
Address

IMPORTANT CONTACTS

Name
Phone
Email
Address

Name
Phone
Email
Address

Name
Phone
Email
Address

Name
Phone
Email
Address

Name
Phone
Email
Address

Name
Phone
Email
Address

Name
Phone
Email
Address

Name
Phone
Email
Address

Made in the USA
Monee, IL
12 November 2026

e65515be-27e5-431e-aac9-d47d2ea3bbc7R02